Several years ago  providence He saw ... to have the youth pastors take me to lunch after ministering in the morning service. It was here I met Danrey and Christie Amoyo. I can still remember the hollow sound that came from Christie as she told me they had no other children, and in fact they had been told by doctors she couldn't have any more children. I felt my entire being come alive within me, and with a bold confidence from the Holy Spirit I said to Christie, "Look at me." I knew at that moment I was carrying a word from heaven. I said to her, "You will have another child! Furthermore, you will have multiple children!" Like Mary, Christie grabbed a hold of that word with her entire being. Over the last couple of years, my wife Gayle and I have had the God-given opportunity to get to know Pastors Danrey and Christie Amoyo. We clearly see the hand of God on their lives.

—Scott and Gayle Willis
Encounter the Flame Ministries
Cincinnati, Ohio

Christie's strength through faith gave her the ability to open up her heart to the risk of having more children after experiencing three miscarriages. Her determination to grow her family after enduring such loss had a direct impact on my life, having gone through my own painful experiences of miscarriage and premature birth. Without Christie's guiding example, I would not have found the strength or courage to persevere in growing my own family, blessing me with two additional beautiful babies here with me today.

—Jennifer Stefansson
Friend and Sister-In-Law

I've known Christie for over ten years, from my teenage years to now as a new mom. Through fellowship, prayer, and sharing scriptures, Christie has helped me through my personal life, and especially with my own pregnancy. Every mom and soon-to-be mom needs to hear Christie's testimony. She is a remarkable example of how keeping God in the centre of your life, the power of prayer, and believing by faith will move mountains. The beautiful family she has today is nothing short of a God-given miracle and an inspiration to all.

—Jamellah Paggao
Friend and Member of Today's Church

Christie has always been a mentor of mine. In 2010 when my husband Rob and I got married, we tried getting pregnant right away with no success. During those hard times, she told me to focus on the positive things and be around positive people who would lift us up. She also listened to God and passed on a fasting book to me in 2012 that completely changed my outlook on praying, giving, and fasting. It was then that we had our first miracle baby girl, Alexis, and two years later our second miracle, baby boy Tobias.

—Sheryll Adriaenssens
Friend and Member of Today's Church

As Christie's cousin, I've watched her grow from a shy little girl to a bold and vivacious woman of God! The biggest change I have seen, however, was when she really grabbed hold of the Word of God and His promises, and cast aside what the world would say in her situation. This especially rang true when it came to her pregnancies. I have cried with her over lost babies and rejoiced with her over the children she now has. The promises of God are yes and amen! Christie's life is a living testimony of that.

—Sue Murdock
Friend and Cousin

The Promised Child

When God Answers Your Prayers in One Area, He Can Do It in Every Area!

The Promised Child

Christie Amoyo

THE PROMISED CHILD
Copyright © 2018 by Christie Amoyo

All rights reserved. Neither this publication nor any part of this publication may be reproduced or transmitted in any form or by any means, electronic or mechanical, including photocopying, recording or any information storage and retrieval system, without permission in writing from the author.

This book is intended to provide helpful information on the subjects discussed, and is not a substitution for medical advice. As in all matters of health, please consult a physician before undertaking any changes to diet, exercise, and medication.

All Scripture quotations, unless otherwise indicated, are taken from the Holy Bible, New International Version®, NIV®. Copyright ©1973, 1978, 1984, 2011 by Biblica, Inc.™ Used by permission of Zondervan. All rights reserved worldwide. www.zondervan.com The "NIV" and "New International Version" are trademarks registered in the United States Patent and Trademark Office by Biblica, Inc.™ Scripture quotations taken from the Amplified® Bible (AMPC), Copyright © 1954, 1958, 1962, 1964, 1965, 1987 by The Lockman Foundation. Used by permission. www.Lockman.org. Scripture quotations marked (NLT) are taken from the Holy Bible, New Living Translation, copyright ©1996, 2004, 2007, 2013, 2015 by Tyndale House Foundation. Used by permission of Tyndale House Publishers, Inc., Carol Stream, Illinois 60188. All rights reserved. Scripture quotations are from the ESV® Bible (The Holy Bible, English Standard Version®), copyright © 2001 by Crossway, a publishing ministry of Good News Publishers. Used by permission. All rights reserved. Scripture quotations marked (KJV) are taken from the Holy Bible, King James Version, which is in the public domain.

Printed in Canada

ISBN: 978-1-4866-1649-7

Word Alive Press
119 De Baets Street, Winnipeg, MB R2J 3R9
www.wordalivepress.ca

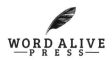
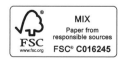

Cataloguing in Publication may be obtained through Library and Archives Canada

Dedication

I want to dedicate this book to my beautiful faith children here on earth—Daniel, Dominic, Cali, and Donovan—and to my children in heaven. One day we will all be together.

I also dedicate this to my amazing husband Danrey, who held my hand and children every step of the way, and who backed me up in love and faith.

To my family and friends, who saw firsthand the struggles and the miracles.

To our good friends, the Willises and Keesees, who listened to God and birthed faith in us. We are forever grateful.

To God, who is the Author and Finisher of our faith.

Contents

1.	The Announcement	1
2.	Daniel	9
3.	Heartbeat	13
4.	Christmas	21
5.	The Promise	25
6.	Our New Reality	33
7.	More to Believe	39
8.	Surprise	45
9.	Full House	53
	Conclusion	61

chapter one
The Announcement

My husband and I met in Bible college and got married when I was twenty-one and he was twenty-two. He grew up in a Christian home whereas I invited Christ into my heart at age two, and then again at age thirteen. But I actually got serious about God at nineteen.

After four years of marriage, my husband and I thought that starting a family was the next step in our lives. We both laughed at the thought of having a whole basketball team of children, but we figured we should just start with one.

We were very busy people. My husband was a youth pastor, worship leader, and young adults pastor, and I joined him in all of it. I also had a full-time job. We both enjoyed sports on the side as well. At that time, we owned our very first home, a small six-hundred-square-foot house. It had two bedrooms and a good yard for our dog. We were twenty-five years old and had our whole exciting life ahead of us.

I was a healthy young woman. I was very active and didn't smoke, drink, or do anything out of the ordinary. One day, my mothering instincts began to kick in and I wanted a baby. I started to watch a lot of mom shows and read up on all sorts of baby topics. I wanted to make sure I knew what I was getting myself into. I wanted to get my body prepared, and I hoped to be one of those moms who would still play sports well into their pregnancy.

The Promised Child

Then the day came when I was late!

I was so excited to rush to my doctor's office, even though I was only a few days late with my period. She took a test for me and said it was faintly positive! She began to prep me about my next appointments and asked me how I was feeling so far. I mentioned that I was experiencing some dizziness. She just told me that dizziness can happen with pregnancy, with my blood flowing to the baby.

Following the appointment, my husband and I went next door to the Chinese food buffet to celebrate. We planned how we were going to tell our parents. We imagined what their reactions would be.

We couldn't keep it to ourselves, even for a few days. We told our family right away and soon enough our circle of friends all knew, even though we hadn't told them yet. News spread quickly.

I was at home doing laundry one day, by myself, when I bent down to pull the dry clothes from the machine. I felt something. Turns out I bled a little bit. I called my grandmother right away so she could pray over me. Then I just took it easy and sat on the couch the rest of the day. I thought maybe I had been doing too much and just needed a rest.

I was only about five and a half weeks along when I noticed some more bleeding. After asking a few people what they thought, I decided that it might be a good idea to get checked. Since it was the weekend, we went to the emergency room. After waiting in the hospital many hours, I got checked out by the doctor and he took some blood tests. He asked if I was having any cramping, but all I had was some pain on my left side, like ovulating pain.

The results said I was pregnant. He didn't think I was miscarrying, but he told me to come back on Monday for another blood

The Announcement

test to make sure my pregnancy hormone levels were rising properly. We went back home, tired and a little confused.

Everyone knew I had been to the emergency room and was concerned about the pregnancy. I didn't know how to react. I was barely pregnant and everything was so new to me.

Monday came around and I took some more blood tests. The tests showed that my hormone levels weren't rising like they were supposed so, so the doctors sent me for an ultrasound. On Wednesday, I returned for this awkward procedure during which the technician told me she didn't even think I was pregnant because she couldn't find a baby.

I was sent home with instructions to check in with my regular doctor once she received the ultrasound results.

I spent the next few days around the house, unable to go to work. I was in some pain still, but I was more scared and confused than anything.

Unfortunately, my parents had gone on vacation at this time and we were house-sitting for them. Since my mom wasn't around, one of my aunts checked in on me. She told me a story about her fallopian tube rupturing while she was pregnant, sending her to the hospital. She prayed with me and hoped that wouldn't be the case for me.

The next evening, my husband came home late and found me doubled over on the living room sofa. I had so much pain on my left side that I could barely walk. We went to the nearest hospital, different from the first one. They unfortunately gave me a bit of a hard time because they had none of my records. The nurses listened to my story and could see the pain I was in. They took blood and saw that

The Promised Child

my hormone levels didn't match up with being seven weeks pregnant. As this was once again the weekend, they told me to come back the following Monday so they could perform an ultrasound.

My parents came home early from their trip so Mom could be there with me at the hospital. We went in Monday and I had the most painful ultrasound. There was the baby, still attached to my left ovary and in my fallopian tube. It was an ectopic pregnancy. The doctors calmly explained that I would not be able to go home; I would need to be operated on because my tube could rupture and I could die.

And there was no way to save the baby.[1]

I hated needles, I hated hospitals, and I was in utter disbelief that I was going in for an emergency operation. As they prepped me, two young student doctors came in and explained my options. They told me that the baby was a little too big now for them to recommend taking a pill that would flesh everything out, but we could still try it. Or I could have the operation. I was already in so much pain, and I knew I would lose the baby. I just wanted this nightmare over, so I chose the operation. The male doctor told me I wouldn't be able to wear a bikini anymore, because I would have a long scar across my abdomen. I just laughed.

They told me that the operation would begin in about an hour. My mom took all the nail polish off my toes and we ended up waiting for about five hours. Then I was wheeled on my bed through the long, dark hallways to the operating rooms. Many times different doctors came in to explain what was going to happen to me.

---

1 I tear up as I write this. It brings back so many emotions.

The Announcement

Then they put the hairnet on me and wheeled me through a set of double doors. The first thing I noticed was the cross above the door. I began to feel so scared and alone. Death didn't cross my mind, though. I wouldn't let it.

"Count back from ten," the doctor said to me. My arm got really hot. I'm sure I passed out at seven.

♥

My husband met me in the recovery room over two hours later, but I don't remember him being there. I just remember crying and hearing myself moan in pain.

When I came to, I couldn't come to terms with what I had just been through. It was all so surreal. I had a huge bandage on my belly and I remember thinking that I would have to look at this mark for the rest of my life.

My doctor ran into the room every now and then to check on how I was healing. Never did he say anything to me, though. The student doctors came to visit me again, too, and they told me it was a good thing they had operated on me because I'd had a lot of blood trapped inside, and it had all needed to come out. They also told me that I was now missing part of my ovary and fallopian tube; the scar tissue could increase my chances of having another ectopic pregnancy.

My mother-in-law worked at the same hospital, which was great. She taught me how to walk again. That might sound silly, but when your abdomen is cut it takes a while to relearn how to use those muscles. I also reacted negatively to every medication they gave me. I was one hundred percent helpless and hopeless.

The Promised Child

Before I was released, a hospital chaplain came to visit. It was nice to pray with someone who was there specifically to help in that terrible situation.

I was sent home a few days later, and then reality set in. I didn't feel up to talking with anyone and I didn't feel like getting out of bed. I was on some heavy medications which probably confused my body and assisted in sending me back to the emergency room days later. I had been sent home with a bladder infection that became severe and made my body really sick.

Now that I was topped up on medication, I did finally start to recover. I had a big bandage on my tummy and had to nurse my wounds. I also lost about fifteen pounds. It was hard to even look in the mirror, never mind have visitors over.

So now what? I thought. My brain had a hard time thinking about it, analyzing every detail. I just wanted to forget it all.

I received many phone calls and much support from my family and friends. Many told me that these things just happened to some people. I

> I JUST KNEW THAT BEING THE WIFE OF A PASTOR DIDN'T PLACE ME ABOVE ANYONE ELSE.

hated that answer. But what I hated even more was a phone call I received from a lady at my church. She asked me, "Why would this happen to you? You are a pastor's wife."

Wow. She actually stumped me on that one. I didn't have any answers. I just knew that being the wife of a pastor didn't place me above anyone else. God wouldn't answer my prayers over others's.

I was really troubled in my spirit because of that question. Did people expect more from a pastor's wife? I spent many days in recovery reading and asking God why these things had happened to me. Why would these things happen to anyone?

I knew the healing process would take a while, and my doctor told me to wait about three months before trying to get pregnant again. She also told me that when I did, it would help to put the whole ectopic pregnancy experience behind me. At that point, I wasn't even sure if I wanted to get pregnant again.

Within a few days, I received a call from a good friend of mine. She was one of the young adult women at church and we spent much time together. She had three children and she'd had a really tough time with her last delivery. Well, she called me because she was in the hospital; even though the doctors had told her not to get pregnant again, she was pregnant. The doctors were now telling her that this pregnancy could kill her and her baby. She wanted me to come and see her and pray for her. I told her I would come.

I got off the phone with her and told God I couldn't do it. This was just too soon for me to try and help anyone else, especially with pregnancy issues.

But I couldn't ignore my friend's plea of. I pushed my feelings aside and went to her bedside.

I prayed with her and talked her through everything. I didn't know exactly how to encourage her, but God put a song in my heart and we just sang a worship song together.

The doctors decided that they had to end the pregnancy. She was so grateful that I could be there with her.

Little did I know that God was healing me as I was helping to heal her.

I took quite a few weeks off from church, because it was really hard to hear everyone's comments there. Hugs and acknowledgement were good, but comments about trying again and God having greater plans were neither good nor helpful.

My husband and I decided it was a good time to take a holiday, so we left the city and went on a secluded vacation. We needed to reconnect and get in touch with each other and enjoy life.

chapter two

Daniel

AFTER THREE MONTHS PASSED, WE ACTUALLY WANTED TO TRY AGAIN. We ended up getting pregnant that first month, and although I was a bit nervous about how the pregnancy would go, I was excited, too. My family doctor had told me that having an ectopic pregnancy was extremely rare, one in a million, and there was almost no chance of us ever having another one. Even though the hospital doctors had told me otherwise, I was optimistic.

We also decided to sell our little home. We were very thankful that it sold for the top price and we were able to pay off some school debts. We felt like we were getting our lives in order and were excited for our future.

We ended up moving in with my parents for a bit while we looked for our new home.

I noticed that I was really nauseous even the first day of having my late period—a good sign. The doctors got me in for an ultrasound at six weeks so they could see if the baby was planted in the proper spot. The baby showed up on the ultrasound, right in the spot where he was supposed to be. I was ecstatic. We told our families right away and everyone just told me to take it easy this time, to get some good rest and not overexert myself. Although some of this advice was helpful, it made me feel like the first pregnancy had been my fault.

The Promised Child

I was extra cautious the first few months of this pregnancy. I did everything by the book. I read all the books about pregnancy again, and everything I experienced this time was exactly as the books said.

After three months, the nausea left completely and I was able to enjoy being pregnant. I ate well, did lots of walking, and only gained twenty-five pounds.

I really enjoyed living with my mom, too. A lot of healing had happened in me and being there was a great support.

One night, I had a stomach-ache and thought it was because of something I'd eaten. While running back and forth to the washroom that night, I noticed that I was doing it every five minutes. I began to keep track, and then it started happening every two minutes. I woke my husband up and told him that I might be in labour. I was about two weeks early.

> IT MADE ME FEEL LIKE THE FIRST PREGNANCY HAD BEEN MY FAULT.

I'd heard so many stories about false labour that I didn't want to go to the hospital at 2:00 in the morning if the doctors were just going to send me home. My husband told me to go wake up my mom, because she would know. I snuck upstairs and woke her up, and once she saw the look on my face when a cramp came she knew it was time!

We grabbed my hospital bag and took off in the night.

After checking in, I was four and a half centimetres dilated. The nurses started hooking me up to all sorts of machines and said I wouldn't be sent home: I was in labour.

Daniel

I felt relieved, but then the pain came on pretty strong. I had watched some natural birth videos prior to all this and thought I would be tough and not need any painkillers or an epidural. I held out as long as I could, and I remember the nurse telling me to start walking the halls because I wasn't dilating fast enough. My husband grabbed my arm to help me up and I told him he could go walk the halls by himself. The pain and fatigue was getting to me.

As soon as they put me in my own delivery room, I took their offer of the epidural. It sounded like a good choice to me. I lay there eating popsicles and watching the bedside machine track my contractions. My husband napped in the chair beside me.

Finally, after thirteen hours and the doctor inducing me and breaking my water, our baby Daniel was born. He was perfect in every way.

Many of the doctors and nurses asked if I had already had a child by caesarean, because of the scar on my abdomen. This brought back memories, but it made me even more grateful to hold my little baby boy. Having him definitely brought much healing after our loss.

We began to raise our precious little boy. He brought so much joy to everyone around him. He was the first grandson for four of his five grandparents.

And now we were parents! Our home filled with laughter and tears as we shopped for cute baby stuff and took so many pictures. You don't realize how much love you have inside you until you have a child. It really helped me connect and understand just how much God loves us. It's wonderful to look at the world through the eyes of a child.

chapter three
Heartbeat

WE MOVED OUT OF MY PARENTS'S HOME WHEN DANIEL WAS A YEAR old. We had fun making up our new home with three bedrooms and a nice little yard.

When Daniel was about a year and a half, we thought it was a good time to grow our family. We were ready to get pregnant once again.

My grandmother had had twins and I was pretty sure that could happen to me, too. So when I did get pregnant again, I was really excited to notice that my belly seemed to be growing quickly. Because I wasn't very nauseous at the beginning and I had some pains in my side, I spoke to my doctor. She couldn't get me in for an ultrasound for a few weeks, but after I hit the seven-week mark and wasn't bleeding I figured we had nothing to worry about.

One day after church, we had a youth group meeting at our house. One of the girls mentioned to me how big my belly was getting, saying that I looked about four months already; I totally agreed. During that meeting, I felt a strong urge to have a cup a tea. I felt like I needed to relax. In fact, as soon as everyone left, I lay down in my bed.

I was extremely nauseous for the following days. I just attributed it to being pregnant, since not all pregnancies are the same. I was eating constantly to get rid of the nausea, trying everything in the book to help me out.

At ten weeks, I finally had an ultrasound appointment. When we went in, my cousin and her husband were in the waiting room as well. We were super excited to see each other and talk about our pregnancies.

Once I was called into the room, everything on the ultrasound monitor looked great to me. I even saw the baby planted in the right spot. When the technician called my husband into the room, I showed him the baby. We both smiled.

Next, the doctor came in and started to examine me.

"How many weeks are you?" he asked.

I told him I was ten weeks, and he explained that the baby was only measuring seven and a half weeks. My heart sank. And then he told us that our baby didn't have a heartbeat.

I broke. I don't even know what he said after that. I was numb.

The doctor told me to get dressed and the technician said that I would have to be admitted. They would have to remove the foetus that very same day.

The moment I left the room, I encountered my cousin in the hallway. Before I could say anything, she saw from my expression that something was wrong. I burst into tears and told her that my baby didn't have a heartbeat, that I would have to stay at the hospital to have a D&C (dilation and curettage). I asked her to notify my family.

As we got to the right floor and checked ourselves in at the admittance desk, I was still tearing up and could barely write my name. After the papers were filled out, the clerk, who I know was trying to be kind, told me to try and have a nice day. I was so shocked she said this to me that I immediately stopped crying.

My husband grabbed me and said, "No, she doesn't mean it!"

It was the worst day. I felt totally beside myself.

I got to my room and thought, *Here we go again.*

My OB/GYN was there that day and came to see me right away. She briefed me on what was going to happen.

"Don't worry," she said. "These things happen sometimes. Soon it will be over and you can try again." She added that she would try to get me in for the procedure as soon as possible.

Well, because I had snacked on half of a peanut butter sandwich that morning, the doctors couldn't perform the procedure for a couple more hours. As I settled into my bed to wait, my husband and I were able to talk and pray together. I began to feel at peace and recall some of the not-so-good symptoms I had been feeling. When someone miscarries, they usually begin to bleed and eventually the foetus does come out. But in my case, my body didn't expel anything. I guess that was why I'd started to get sick, tired, and nauseated. I remembered the day when we'd had people over and all I had wanted was tea and a nap. That was the day, I believe, that my baby's heart stopped.

This time, we got an immediate visit from the hospital chaplain. We had a nice talk and told her we had been in this situation before. She notified us of a service they have for all those who have lost babies. We would be getting an invitation to attend.

My husband called our families to let them know where we were and what was going on. My mother planned to bring our son Daniel to visit us; he missed his mommy. I turned my thoughts to

The Promised Child

how precious my son was. This greatly comforted me. It didn't take them long to arrive. The moment Daniel came into my room, he got up on the bed and took his shoes off. He snuggled right up to me, almost like he was thinking, *If Mom's here, then I'm here, too.*

A few hours passed and my family went home. My husband went to the gift store on the main floor and bought us a little checkers game to pass the time.

In the evening, my doctor came in. "Don't worry. We will get you in before the day is over."

At 11:30 p.m., she finally came into my room and told me it was my turn. Again they put the hairnet on me and wheeled me to the operating room. I saw the same cross on the door and the many people in the room waiting for me to arrive. My arm began to burn and I passed out.

It was about 12:30 when I got back to my room. I remember waking up and being so hungry. The nurse gave me juice and a sandwich, which satisfied me for a moment. But then it came back up and out. She got me to take it easy for a little bit, then sent us home at 1:30 in the morning. What a day.

The next days at home were terribly quiet. I really had no words to say. This time I felt like I'd been a lot farther along and everyone had known I was pregnant. I was okay talking with people this time, but I didn't want to talk about *it*. I didn't want to go there. I hid a lot of my pain and tried to act strong. But I really didn't know how to come to terms with everything. I was still a pastor's wife. Why would these things happen to me?

Heartbeat

A lady in my church came up to me the Sunday I got back, and in passing she put her hand near my tummy and loudly asked if I was pregnant. During the service later, I sat and played it over in my head. I'd just wanted to run away. She hadn't even known I had been pregnant. That had felt like a punch in the gut.

> I HID A LOT OF MY PAIN AND TRIED TO ACT STRONG.

In the following weeks, I planned a surprise birthday party for my husband at our house. He would be coming home to our family and friends. While I was setting things up, he came home early and realized what I was doing. He's really not the surprise party type.

About an hour before the guests were to come, I buckled over in pain in my kitchen. My husband quickly came and I told him that I just needed to lie down for a moment. I felt stabbing pains in my left ovary—pains I recognized.

After a few minutes of lying down, the pain subsided and I figured I would get up and help with the party. But when I stood, I could tell that my body had just gotten rid of something down there. I bled quite a bit. An oval shape, just larger than a quarter, came out of me. I wrapped it up and got my sister-in-law to drive me to the hospital.

I felt really bad leaving my husband to host his own party, but I didn't know what else to do. We got to the hospital and had to wait a few hours before I could be seen. When I did go in, the nurses couldn't wrap their minds around my story. All they said about what had come out of me was that it was definitely a tissue mass. They couldn't confirm anything else, so they sent me home.

The Promised Child

They informed my OB/GYN on the following Monday, though, and she quickly called me for an appointment. She didn't know what it could have been, either, except that she was sure she had gotten everything out during the D&C.

My conclusion was that this could have been the twin. It's possible that one baby had gotten stuck in my fallopian tube while the second one had been planted properly. But neither survived.

Here I was in recovery mode again. But this time I had a little boy I could focus my time and energy on. I was so thankful for him.

Not too long after all this, I got a call from a good friend of mine, a non-Christian girl with whom I had never talked about God. But she had just miscarried and needed to talk to me.

"Is my baby in heaven?" she asked me.

Wow. I was the only one she could talk to at this time, since no one close to her had ever been in her situation. As we spoke, I was able to encourage her.

I knew God was bringing healing to me again. Whatever we sow, we shall reap.

It took a really long time to get over this loss. I found myself not wanting to go out a lot. I preferred to sleep or stay in the house than anything else besides work. I felt like I had lost all hope of ever getting pregnant again.

I now know that I was dipping into depression, although I didn't recognize it at the time. Looking back, I recognize those feelings, those thoughts, those actions; I was starting to go down a slippery slope.

At that time, my husband and I weren't too close in our relationship. Life seemed hard in every area, which just added to the pain. I would hide all my pain and frustration until it burst out of me. Little did I know that men deal with their own burden—the high expectations that life and family can put on them. Our lives were a bit messy.

Still, many people often asked us, "When are you going to have another baby?"

We received an invitation to join the memorial service the hospital held for all those who had lost their babies. It happened on a nice summer day and our parents joined us for the small ceremony. It was actually quite healing to hear them call out "Amoyo babies." We hadn't been able to go to our first baby's memorial, so we remembered all of them this time.

It was nice that the hospital recognized our losses, and it was eye-opening to see so many other families there. We all connected on a deep level.

chapter four

Christmas

We weren't sure if we were going to try again for a baby. I felt like I could come to terms with an ectopic pregnancy and why it had failed, but I had a hard time understanding why my last baby hadn't had a heartbeat. That felt completely uncontrollable. What if something bad happened again? I hated to think about this. My heart felt so broken about it all.

But we did really want another baby and decided to try just one more time.

Almost one year later, I found myself pregnant again, just before Christmas. I was quite surprised that it took so much longer this time. When we told our family and close friends, there wasn't too much excitement. It was hard, even for us, to get excited. People told us not to spread the news just yet and to wait until we knew for sure that everything was going to be okay.

I didn't have any nausea or pain, so when I started to bleed on Christmas Eve I felt really disappointed and hopeless. I was only six weeks along. I sat in the ER waiting room, getting mad at God. Of all days, why Christmas? Why me? I just didn't get it.

After my examination, they sent me again for an ultrasound and found that I'd had yet another ectopic pregnancy. The only good thing about it this time was that it looked like my body was trying to get rid of everything. I prayed that I wouldn't have to go through another D&C. I just wanted to go home to my son.

When the emergency room doctor came to see me, he bent down, looked me right in the eyes, and asked me if I understood that this was a failing pregnancy. With tears in my eyes, I nodded. He told me that he was sorry. That was the first time I really felt the heart of a doctor. He cared for what I was going through.

They asked me to come back the following day, Christmas Day, and give a blood sample to make sure that my pregnancy hormone levels were dropping. If they weren't, further measures would have to be taken.

I have no words to describe what that Christmas Eve was like, with all this heartache. I turned my sadness into anger when I realized that I was missing Christmas with Daniel. I wasn't going to let him be affected by this.

We went to my mother's house to pick him up and see the rest of the family who was still there. Then we quietly snuck back to our home.

This was the first time my husband told me that he felt like there was a hole in his stomach. He didn't know how to explain it, but he felt physically empty inside.

For the next five days, I had to go back to the emergency room and give blood. Then my doctor confirmed that it was all over.

I didn't feel like reading the Bible that week, or even praying. I was so hurt and confused. I heard people say, "Maybe they were only meant to have one child" or "God is coming soon. It's probably better this way." I didn't even know what to say to God. I really didn't want to hear that any of those things were true.

After a few weeks of frustration and denial, I had it in my heart to read my daily devotions book. I turned to the correct page and found a scripture reading from Revelation.

Oh great, I thought. *Here we go with the end-of-the-world talk.*

But as I read the scripture, it hit me so deep: *"You are worthy, our Lord and God, to receive glory and honor and power, for you created all things, and by your will they were created and have their being"* (Revelation 4:11, NIV). I immediately felt like God was speaking these words right to me: "Don't worry. I created your babies and I have them with me." God had wanted to create them, and now they were with Him.

I thought about that word for weeks, and I was able to share it with others who had lost their babies, too. I need to share with others what God was revealing to me after all the failed pregnancies. Many women needed to hear it.

> GOD HAD WANTED TO CREATE THEM, AND NOW THEY WERE WITH HIM.

No one had talked to me before about this aspect of wanting a family. It was extremely difficult not having anyone to talk to. I needed someone who understood my physical and emotional pain, but also God's part in it. Although I didn't have all the answers, what I did know helped me to help others. I became the one person others could go to when they needed comfort and understanding.

My husband and I decided that we weren't going to try to have another baby. We wanted to get on with our lives, and I ended up getting a new job. It was time to move on and focus on raising our little superstar, Daniel.

chapter five
The Promise

SOMETHING HAPPENED ABOUT SIX MONTHS AFTER WE MADE THE decision not to try growing our family anymore. One day at church we had a guest pastor come and speak. Well, he not only preached the Word, but he did it with tremendous fire and started to lay hands on people. People were falling all over the floor. The power of the Holy Spirit was overwhelming. I remember thinking, *Who is this guy? He's a Christian, like me, but I don't act like this.* I was so amazed at this anointing, and I didn't know why we, and our church, didn't act like this.

When the service was over, our pastor was busy, so he asked my husband and I to take that guest pastor out for lunch. We were so excited to just be able to hang out with our new friend, Pastor Scott Willis. We wanted to know where he came from and about this anointing and power he walked in.

When we got to the restaurant, as we waited for our table, he asked us the dreaded question: "You have only one child. Are you going to have more?"

I thought he was just trying to make small talk with us.

We told him that we had tried many times and had suffered many losses. There was silence.

The Promised Child

As the waitress sat us at our table, Pastor Scott looked over the table at me and stared into my eyes.

"You will have more," he said, speaking right into my soul.

He began to tell me about his daughter-in-law, who had been pregnant with twins and needed to go to the hospital. In the hospital, the doctors told her that one twin had a "messed-up" umbilical cord, which actually meant that one twin hadn't been getting enough blood flow or the nutrients needed to develop. The condition was called twin-to-twin transfusion, and the doctors explained that it wasn't reversible. If the couple didn't take steps to end the pregnancy, the condition would eventually kill both babies.

So the couple took a stand of faith and believed God for the impossible.

Pastor Scott's wife stood outside the hospital room and wouldn't let anyone come inside who was going to speak negative words over the situation.

Not even five minutes after they found out about the situation, Pastor Scott received a call from one of their evangelistic friends who had just been about to start preaching, across the world, when she got a strong Word that she had to call him and tell him that everything was going to be okay. They placed the phone on the daughter-in-law's belly and they all prayed.

After five days of proclaiming God's promise, the doctors came into the room with another ultrasound report. They didn't know how to explain it, but the umbilical cord was now fine and both babies were perfect in size and condition. At first they blamed their misdiagnosis on their machines, but then they agreed that a miracle must have taken place.

Pastor Scott looked right into my eyes again. "You know why I'm telling you this, right?"

I burst into tears. Having another baby was a dream I'd thought I had to let go of. I received that Word into the deepest part of me.

Everyone else showed up for lunch, and then someone else drove Pastor Scott back to his hotel.

My husband and I drove home in silence and wonder. We couldn't believe what had happened. It was unforgettable. Little did I know that faith was birthed that day!

That Word kept penetrating my heart, and I couldn't get it out of my mind.

We got pregnant not too long after, and there was definitely something different with me this time: I just *knew* that everything would be okay. Whenever any fear came into my mind, I thought about Pastor Scott's Word, which I knew God had given him. I believe, to this day, that God sent him for us.

> I RECEIVED THAT WORD INTO THE DEEPEST PART OF ME.

I began to let people know that we were pregnant again, and before they could even say anything I told them not to worry—everything was going to be fine with me and our baby.

I started feeling pain in my left side again, but every time I felt the pain I remembered that Word and I had peace.

Our friends were planning their wedding at this time and it was going to take place in Hawaii. My husband, our son, and I were all a part of their wedding. We were so excited. This would be our first big vacation since we'd gotten married and I had never been

The Promised Child

overseas before. Once as I told my doctor that I was pregnant and going to Hawaii, she set us up with an ultrasound appointment as soon as possible.

I was nauseous and having some pain, so yes, I was a little nervous about the ultrasound. I really had to focus on not stressing out and keep remembering what God had promised.

When we went in, I knew that God had given the technician the words to say: "Your baby is in the right spot and has a very strong heartbeat."

Yep, that's all I needed to hear. I played those words over and over in my head the rest of the day, and I can still hear them. God had confirmed everything. I was so happy and thankful.

We went to Hawaii and had an amazing time.

At this point in our lives, we had been opened up to faith living—not just reading the Bible for encouragement but believing that God wanted to teach us more.

♥

My husband started to work through his own struggles at this time. We could see that our lives weren't lining up with what God talked about. Everything my husband did was in his own strength, which brought on so much stress. He fell into a deep depression and had a lot of anxiety.

The struggle was on. Our marriage was full of frustration most days, and our finances were terrible. We had many on-again, off-again days, moving forward in our faith one day and then stepping backward and feeling like our lives were falling apart. Yet I was pregnant and we knew deep down that it was a miracle.

We ended up selling our house and were able to move into my parents's home again. We wanted to clean up our finances and we really needed their support. Even though I was pregnant, most people weren't sure the baby was going to make it. Even worse, my husband was in and out of the hospital with panic attacks and spent days at a time in bed, depressed.

I tried to make every day enjoyable for our son. It was really hard, because I was emotionless. I didn't want to wallow in pity and tears; I was pregnant and had an amazing blessing growing inside me. I didn't want Daniel to feel any of the stress and become immersed in this emotional rollercoaster we were on. All I could do was stay consistent and pray. I believed in God, and He *would* help us through.

The pregnancy was going great and I was enjoying my new job. Every time I met a doubt or fear, from myself or anyone else, I quickly shut that door by speaking only positively about it and thanking God for my baby.

A friend of mine had read a book about childbirth and photocopied a bunch of pages from it for me to read. It took scriptures from the Bible and showed you how to use them to pray for your baby, every single inch of the baby, and yourself too. It was very encouraging, and I read it over almost daily.

I also had the revelation one day that there is no sickness in heaven; the Lord's Prayer in Matthew 6:10 says, *"[Y]our kingdom come, your will be done, on earth as it is in heaven"* (NIV). I decided that if headaches and heartburn didn't exist in heaven, I didn't need to accept them here on earth either. During this pregnancy, I got major heartburn every single night before bed. So every night I told that heartburn to go in Jesus' name, for heartburn wasn't accepted in heaven. And it would leave. When I got a headache, even when I get them today, I commanded it to go—and I was always reminded then to drink more water. God has every answer.

With my husband going through almost a year of this mental and physical struggle, though, all I could do was pray. I learned that I could choose to encourage or discourage. I knew that God was changing things in my mind when it came to believing His Word, and I always believed that my husband was going to get through this.

One day, he rose up in strength and desired change. He had come across Joyce Meyer's book *Battlefield of the Mind*, and he literally consumed it for weeks. He chose to change his thinking, of himself and his thoughts towards God. This started to heal him.

This change actually brought us to a point in our lives where we became so hungry to listen to what God was revealing to us that we took some time away from serving in the church and just soaked. This literally went on for months. Slowly we started to get back to church and get more involved in our ministries again. But things were definitely different with us.

This time I had nausea the entire pregnancy and I gained forty pounds. All I wanted to do was drink milk and eat perogies. The pregnancy also lasted through the winter, so I didn't get too much exercise.

We prayed that I would have the baby on a Saturday. Then, on a Saturday morning at 8:00 a.m., my water broke. Wow, perfect timing!

This labour was different than my first. The nurses didn't give me any painkillers for a long time and tried to get me to have a hot shower and bounce on an exercise ball… I wasn't happy about any of it. Finally the doctor came in and told the nurses, "Get this lady an epidural already!"

The Promise

The anaesthesiologist was taking a while and I needed something now, so they gave me fentanyl. They only gave me half of the dose, and because my head spun they decided not to give me anymore. When they finally came in to give me the epidural, I was relieved. But it didn't have time to kick in fully before my labour started to advance. Only a short while later, I was ready to push.

The doctor came in and warned me that there would be lots of stinging. That scared me. And he was right. My baby's shoulders didn't want to come out, and he was literally like a purple little football when he was born. He was a big little boy.

I unfortunately didn't get to keep him in the room right away. Because of the fentanyl, he had to get checked over. That's not a choice I recommend to anyone.

After ten hours of labour, my beautiful promised child Dominic was born. We cried so much. God's promise and our dream had come true.

chapter six
Our New Reality

SOMEONE ONCE SAID TO US, "THERE'S FAITH, AND THEN THERE'S reality." Well, I want to tell you that faith *is* reality.

After having Dominic, we couldn't stop telling people what God had done in our lives. Dominic was the promise that was born. I had him. I could hold him. He wasn't just a thought or a wish; he was here with us.

My husband came out of his horrible pit of depression and anxiety, because he, too, now believed in God for more. Financially, though, we were just barely getting by, and my parents decided to move out of their house and let us rent it from them. This was great, but we hadn't figured out our financial solution yet. We greatly desired to learn and believe God for that! He had already healed our bodies in so many ways; we figured he cared about our finances, too.

We really started to change our mindsets to believe and trust that God wanted to be more in our lives. We listened to some preachers on television and were amazed to hear their testimonies. We desired to live the blessed life that Pastor Robert Morris talked about.

One day, my mom received some CDs in the mail. She had ordered Pastor Gary Keesee's *Revolution 2.0*, and she thought we would like to have them. The day she gave them to us, we were headed to a church family camp. In fact, we had left our house with no money and our cable had just been cut off. Sigh. That doesn't make you feel too good when you're heading out of town with your toddler and baby. We couldn't even use our credit card; it was maxed out.

My husband had been asked by his parents to speak at this family camp, so we assumed we could ask them for gas money to get home. And our lodging and food would be provided for the next few days. Getting out of town sounded pretty great with everything that was going on.

Camp was only about forty-five minutes away and we agreed that we would try to

> THE FAITH TESTIMONIES AND BLESSED LIFE WE HAD HEARD ABOUT WERE ACTUALLY ATTAINABLE.

listen to this new CD set from my mom. We popped in part one and were *blown away*. Everything Pastor Gary spoke about was exactly what we had gone through—what we were presently going through. Then he spoke a series of Kingdom principles that totally revolutionized our minds! We just knew that God had a greater plan than we knew. The faith testimonies and blessed life we had heard about were actually attainable.

In fact, my husband was so excited about this teaching that he decided to speak about it at camp. We had only finished the first CD by the time we made it to camp, and we couldn't wait to drive home again so we could listen to the next one.

We made a commitment to God, right there, that we wanted to learn everything we could about this faith life and live it out. Our passion had been ignited when we heard the faith testimonies. Faith had already been spoken into our lives, and these CDs gave us the understanding behind it all. These miracles in our lives weren't just

Our New Reality

a result of God finally answering some of our prayers; they were the *evidence* of our faith. We believed, we stood on the Word, and we expected God to move!

On the very last day of camp, we received a financial gift from the group that was there. We were really excited to receive it and start this new faith walk with Christ, and our new understanding of His Kingdom. But it didn't end there. A couple from the group that was heading out early came to give us a larger financial gift of their own. They spoke great encouragement from what my husband had preached about.

God was encouraging us, blessing us, and confirming what was birthing in us. It was so exciting! We were beside ourselves as we left the camp. We went home with enough to tithe, with thankful hearts, pay for gas, and cover our cable bill. We popped in the next CD on the way home and ate up every word of it!

> WE LEARNED HOW TO BELIEVE AND WALK IN FAITH AND SEE ACTUAL RESULTS.

We spent the next few months consumed with those CDs. We listened to them over and over and started to implement the things we were learning. People began to take notice of the way we conducted our actions, as well as our talk. It wasn't like we were out of our financial issues right then and there, but we weren't stressed out about them anymore. We weren't stressed out about our health anymore, either. We learned how to believe and walk in faith and see actual results.

God answers every prayer every time. He loves us. It may not be in the exact way you think He should do it, but you just have to trust and speak what you're expecting!

The Promised Child

Our friends wanted to know what was going on with us, so we invited them over and let them hear our CDs, too. Our friends were so excited to hear them that some of them didn't even want to leave our house. We were a bunch of young adults who really wanted to share what God was doing. Their hearts and minds were also revolutionized.

My husband and I tried to implement some of the things we were learning into our ministries at church. Unfortunately, it just wasn't something we could teach freely about, and our lives couldn't deny that God was up to something. We had a fear about getting people's hopes up. Maybe God wouldn't answer their prayers like He had ours.

For many years, my grandmother had said that we would have our own church one day. We just laughed and took it as a compliment. But it was now impressed on our hearts to share this new truth with our friends, family, and whoever needed to hear how our lives were changing—and it was so simple. God doesn't make things difficult. We do.

My husband wasn't sure what to think or do about all these thoughts yet... until he received a dream. In the dream, God wrote the words "Today's Church" in large bold letters in front of him. That was all he remembered when he woke up.

He was hesitant to tell me about the dream at first. We already had the desire within us to share the message, so now that he'd had a vision it was time to do something about it.

One night when our friends came over to hear the last session of the CDs, we let them know what God was impressing on our hearts. We wanted to warn them that we weren't going to be around

Our New Reality

the church much longer because we would be starting our own ministry. To our surprise, most of them looked at us and said that they were coming, too. Everything we had been sharing with them was changing their lives and they couldn't deny that the changes were mind-blowing and exciting. One friend even threw her first seed money at us and told us that it was for *our* ministry. Faith was arising!

We didn't know how to start a church, nor did we have the finances backing up our decision, but we easily found a venue and paid the rent for the first Sunday. Our parents backed up our decision, too, and many family members came who had once said, "If you ever start a church, we will be there."

To our surprise, that was also the start of another pregnancy. God was definitely taking us farther, faster in our faith. We had to learn and gain wisdom quickly. We stayed in very close fellowship with the eight people who came with us. They spoke faith and encouragement to us. We were all strengthened by the Word and by each other.

In just a few short months, my husband and I purchased my parents's home, drastically cleaning up our finances. As Pastor Gary Keesee often says, "When you take care of the money thing, you can have vision." That's totally what was happening. We weren't worried every day about provision; that's what blocks many people's vision. We trusted God and saw results.

Being able to bless and help others was the life we wanted. We could see all our friends and family being stretched and starting to dream for themselves again, too.

The Promised Child

God put it on our hearts to have one Sunday every month devoted to sharing testimonies. It was so encouraging to hear the great things God was bringing so many people out of and into!

chapter seven

More to Believe

As I mentioned, I got pregnant when we started our ministry. We were really excited as a family to add another blessing into this great vision God was bringing forth. This time it seemed easy to stay on track with proclaiming God's promises over the pregnancy, the baby, and my body. Even early on, when I felt little pains in my abdomen, I didn't give them a thought. The more you move in faith, the more confident you become. If God has answered that kind of prayer before, He can do it again.

My OB/GYN wasn't concerned this time around, either. She made my first appointment at the three-month mark, which surprised me. She was pleased with how things were going. At twenty weeks, she sent me for the routine ultrasound. I got to see the baby and everything looked great to me. The technician asked me if we wanted to know the sex, and this time we actually said yes. It was a girl!

We told everyone right away. I was kind of excited to pass on all the boy clothes and buy some girlie ones.

I went in for another check-up a few weeks later. I'm grateful for how professional my OB/GYN was. She knew just how to say things so I wouldn't worry about anything. She really took control of the situation.

The Promised Child

She told me that I would have to go for another ultrasound in a few weeks because they couldn't see the umbilical cord properly and they had to check it out. She also quickly mentioned that they had found a white spot on the baby's heart that could be related to Down syndrome.

Well, that took me by surprise. She said it so quick that I didn't even have time to react or ask questions. I left that appointment and went to our car, where my husband was waiting. I explained to him everything I had been told and added that I didn't accept the white spot as anything; our baby was not going to have Down syndrome.

Please don't take that the wrong way. Children with Down syndrome are beautiful in every way, but something rose up in me and I didn't accept what she was telling me.

We went home and I told my mom what the doctor had said. Immediately she said that the white spot was Jesus' light inside her. I loved that response, and it was the one I thought about for the next five months.

We didn't tell anyone else about this. The more you say something, the more real it becomes.

If you think I wasn't flooded with thoughts or images of what could possibly be wrong with the baby's umbilical cord and white spot, you're wrong. For months, I had to fight my mind and take up the Word concerning these things.

> I HAD TO FIGHT MY MIND AND TAKE UP THE WORD CONCERNING THESE THINGS.

When we went for the next ultrasound, the technician immediately saw the cord properly, and she didn't mention any other concerns.

At this point in our lives, God reminded us of Pastor Scott, who had spoken into our lives previously. We wanted to track him down to thank him. After a few weeks of phone tag, we finally got his cell phone number. That was a bit intimidating! We didn't even know if he would remember us. We just wanted to thank him and tell him about us having more children, just like he had said. We also wanted to tell him how that Word had birthed faith in us, and how that had spread to starting a new church.

One night, we picked up the phone and called. We thought he was two hours earlier than us, but he turned out to be two hours later than us, meaning that we called him at midnight. Whoops! The funny thing is, he was supposed to be away speaking in Africa, but his plans got messed up and he was actually at home. He picked up his phone and immediately remembered who we were. He was so happy to hear from us and our growing family, but he added that he wanted to come to our church. Wow! That was totally something God had set up. Just a few months later, he and his wife came to visit us and they held a service.

That was only the beginning of our great teamwork together.

The pregnancy seemed to go really fast. It was so much fun having a little girl baby shower. Pretty pink things are my favourite. Our baby was blessed!

One of my prayers this time was that the delivery would go quickly. I really didn't want it to be long and painful like the others. We also prayed that it would work out so we wouldn't have to miss a Sunday church service.

The Promised Child

I had been almost two weeks early with both of my other children, so I expected her to arrive in the same timeframe, if not sooner. She was due in December, so I figured the sooner the better.

One particular Sunday, I woke up and just wasn't feeling great. I didn't have the energy to watch my other children at church while my husband preached, and my size was starting to take a toll on me, so I decided to stay home.

When evening came around, my mother was with me at the house. I had bounced on an exercise ball all day long and by now I felt like I was having contractions.

My husband came home around 8:00 p.m. and was surprised to hear that I was having contractions, even though they weren't regular. My mother noticed that I hadn't moved from the awkward position I had been in for the last hour, so I really wasn't sure if I was in labour or not. My mom prepared to spend the night anyway.

About two hours later, my contractions still weren't regular, and not too painful, so I prayed that God would show me if we should go to the hospital or not. A few seconds after that prayer, I ended up having a really strong contraction. That was my confirmation.

When we got to the hospital, there were a few women ahead of me. Because I wasn't contracting regularly, they made me sit in the waiting area. When it was my turn to check in, the contractions became consistent and they brought me to a bed. All the private rooms were filled, so I had to share a room with someone.

Then our nurse came to us and said that she'd seen that we pastored a church and didn't have insurance. She was a believer, too, and offered to get us into a private room. That was such a blessing.

We were so happy about this that my water broke! Then my husband knocked his water on the floor! We started to laugh so hard—in between contractions.

It was the best labour yet. The nurse came in to check me around 12:30 a.m. and noticed that I was advancing quickly. They rushed me into my room. I really didn't know what my delivery nurse was thinking, but she didn't talk to me much and I kept telling her that the contractions weren't stopping. I thanked God that this labour was going quickly, but then I was also trying to pray away the pain.

The nurse tried to give me some gas to take my thoughts off the pain. It didn't work for me. All of a sudden, I told her that I was pushing. I don't think she believed me, because she hadn't even set my bed up properly. She calmly checked me and walked over to her phone and called for some extra nurses. The doctor was busy delivering another baby at that moment.

I was sideways lying down when I just had to push. Within minutes, my baby girl was born. The nurse was so calm delivering her. Later she told me, "By the way, her umbilical was around her neck when she came out, so I just slipped it off." Really?! I believe that if that nurse hadn't been so divinely calm, there could have been a real panic in that delivery room.

> GOD'S PEACE HAD MADE THE WHOLE EXPERIENCE AMAZING.

My baby girl was healthy and strong and beautiful. The doctor arrived and was so impressed with everyone in the room; God's peace had made the whole experience amazing.

The Promised Child

I spent the next full day in hospital, sharing my faith testimonies with three different nurses. They were so encouraged not only to hear but to see my testimonies.

Baby Cali and I went home the following day. I didn't need to have any stitches at all, as my recovery was so quick. I even showed up at church with her the following Sunday.

As I write these words, it's the eve of her third birthday. She has been the happiest little girl—rough and tumble like her brothers now, but a sweet little princess all the same.

chapter eight

Surprise

We felt complete now as a family and our lives were headed in a great direction. Being able to see our prayers answered and our testimony affecting so many people felt absolutely amazing. God was revealing such a great vision to us. Although having three young children can be a handful at times, it's still wonderful. We must appreciate every moment we have.

In our ministry, we took a leap and invited Pastors Gary and Drenda Keesee to come to our church and hold a conference. They were the ones who had revolutionized our minds and showed us how to walk by faith. We desperately wanted to share the way and the Word that had changed our lives.

When they came, it seemed almost surreal that they were having lunch with us, eating, speaking, and even shopping. They got to hear our story and see how much God had done in our lives in such a short while. Drenda encouraged me to write out my pregnancy testimony and send it to her. A few weeks after they left, I sent it to her. Little did I know, they actually talked about us on their television program. She shared our testimonies on TV and regularly point people to us and our church. What a blessing.

I was also focused on the other ministry my husband and I do: sports outreach. He runs basketball leagues and I have a ladies

The Promised Child

volleyball league that continues to grow every year. It's something I really put my heart and effort into. A lot of women join who love to play and I get to pray with them all. They may not know God or go to church, but they get to hear about Him every week and have a safe and fun place to play volleyball.

One particular year, I finally got to play. Running the league took a lot of work and I had been pregnant on and off, so I was really excited to be on a team and actually play a whole season. I tried getting myself into good shape and practiced lots. I knew I was getting older, and after three babies I needed to work a bit harder. I even decided to hire official referees to take the league a step up so I wouldn't have to worry about doing that part myself.

On the first day, the head referee wanted to meet me. He was intrigued that I had called the league Christian Women's Volleyball League. He was a Christian and wondered what I did in this league to make it different. The other referee who came with him wasn't a Christian, and the head referee was so happy to see him join us when it came to praying before each game. I know he caught the vision with me.

Even more amazing, I found out that his wife was the one who had written the book on childbirth that my friend had photocopied for me. What a setup! He was so encouraged to hear about how his wife's book had helped encourage me for my pregnancies.

Our team did great that season and we ended up making it to the championship game. A few days prior, though, I wasn't feeling myself—and I was late. Yep, pregnant again! My husband and I were stunned. This definitely hadn't been in our plans. We were really happy, though!

Surprise

It was just before Mother's Day when we found out, so when we took our mothers out for lunch we told them that their gift wasn't coming until December. They and the rest of the family were totally surprised. My doctor wasn't surprised, though. She just laughed. She was very happy that we were able to have another baby after all the loss.

But when it came to volleyball, I couldn't dive or play the way I wanted to. My teammates asked what was going on, and I told them. Although we lost the game, they were also very happy for us.

My checkups went well and I again took out all my pregnancy scriptures. The pain and discomfort didn't bother me. I knew everything would be great.

At the ultrasound, it was exciting to see the baby, and this time the technician told me I had to wait to find out the sex. I was so sure that it was another girl, though. This pregnancy felt the same as my last one, and I had already given away all my boy stuff.

Well, the OB/GYN's assistant later called me and said, "It's a boy!"

I was so shocked. It made for a great surprise.

Next, I had to take a test to rule out gestational diabetes. The night before the test, I made a batch of irresistible chocolate chip cookies. Yes, I ate about ten of them, just to make sure they were a good batch. So the next day I ended up failing the test and was asked to fast and come back. Now, I did usually watch what I ate and kept my body healthy, but it was a bit more of a challenge not to indulge my cravings.

My doctor called me when she got the results back. "Christie, because you failed one of the three tests, we now have to send you

The Promised Child

to the diabetic centre for monitoring. If this was last year, one failed test wouldn't matter, but they changed the rules for this year. Sorry."

I begged her to opt out of this, as I thought it was crazy. I'd never had any of these issues with my other babies or pregnancies, but she insisted that I at least meet with the dietician. Sigh. Fine. I decided to go for my doctor's sake.

I entered the diabetic centre and had to fill out an information page before I met with anyone. The first line on it asked, "How long have you had diabetes for?" I wrote, "I do not have diabetes." That question alone was enough to push my buttons.

Not only had I experienced many healings, I had prayed for people to receive healings. I had seen too much. God has already provided healing for us. If we fully convince ourselves of this, and if we can get that promise and the Word inside of us, we can all move mountains. Anyway, I've learned to fight the good fight of faith and I won't let anyone tell me that I'm sick in any way whatsoever.

I was called into a room to meet the dietician. She was really a sweet girl who told me everything I already knew about the foods I should and shouldn't eat. It was a good reminder to think about these things regularly and check my diet. But when she pulled out a little machine to check my blood sugar three times a day, I told her no. I wasn't willing to do that. I told her I didn't have diabetes and I didn't plan on having it.

> WE CAN ALL MOVE MOUNTAINS.

But I humoured her. We finally came to an agreement for me to test my blood sugar once a day for the next two weeks.

Surprise

Two weeks later, I returned with the results—and all were extremely normal, except one. That concerned her, which I thought was crazy because she had just finished telling me that even the use of hand soap can affect the test. I tried not to roll my eyes.

She asked me to do another two weeks of testing, and to do it three times at least one day each week. I also had to write in detail everything I was eating and at what times.

I returned again two weeks later. My results were all normal. Then we discussed my previous pregnancies and the weight of my other children at birth. She asked me to email her if I had any concerns over the next couple of weeks.

Oh good, I thought. *That's all over.*

But at my next OB/GYN checkup, the assistant came into the room and handed me a piece of paper with the date and time of a gestational diabetes ultrasound. I asked the assistant why I needed this, and she told me that it was for my gestational diabetes. I told her that I didn't have gestational diabetes, and she just laughed and walked out.

A lot of people probably think I'm crazy, which I understand, but I do not accept any sickness or disease.

My husband and I went to that silly ultrasound appointment feeling a bit annoyed. I am very kind to people, but don't tell me that me or my children or family is sick.

The lady called us in and looked me up and down. I had only gained twenty-five pounds in total and was about to have the baby any day now, so she got me to lie down.

"How long have you had diabetes for?" she asked.

"I do not have diabetes."

The Promised Child

"You failed your test," she snapped back at me. "And now you have diabetes."

I felt the fire stir up inside me.

Next, she told us that my doctor had set up this appointment because she was worried that the baby was going to be too big and could have some serious problems. I looked at my husband and he looked away; he knew I wanted to snap back at her. But I didn't. The awkwardness in the room was thick. I wouldn't argue, just stand my ground.

She quietly gave me the ultrasound and excused herself from the room to go check with the doctor. When she came back into the room, she had a completely different demeanour. She explained that the baby was the perfect size and didn't have anything wrong with him. I was free to go.

Unfortunately, she added, I would have to come in for another ultrasound in two weeks to see again if there had been any changes. I just told her that I would have had the baby by then.

My previous delivery had gone great, so I expected this one to go even better. I was really hoping to have him before Christmas.

But Christmas passed, leaving me feeling anxious. Everyone around me was anxiously waiting as well. My mom had her sleepover bag packed even longer than I had mine.

One early morning I woke up and wasn't sure why, so I went back to sleep.

When I awoke again, at 4:00 a.m., I felt a cramp. But I was so tired that I fell back asleep.

By 4:30, I couldn't put myself back to sleep anymore so I went to the washroom and started to walk around a bit to see if the contractions were regular. I began to time them, and they seemed to be coming every four minutes or so.

I called my mom and got her to come to our house so we could leave for the hospital. My husband, frantic, flew out of bed and ran outside to warm up the van.

At the hospital, I could barely walk or talk properly while the nurses checked me. They rushed me in, as I was already seven centimetres dilated. They knew that my last delivery had only lasted two hours, so this baby was coming soon.

The issue this time was that there wasn't enough time to administer antibiotics for Strep B. My tests had been positive for this, so my husband and I just thanked God that it wasn't going to affect the baby.

I progressed very quickly, with a lot of nurses stepping in and out of my room, banging my bed into position. My water hadn't broken yet, though, which everyone was waiting for. It seemed really hectic this time, and it didn't help that the doctor came in and started almost yelling at me to get into a better position. He was really negative about the fact that I couldn't do everything he asked me to do. That just made me kind of stressed. I had to keep focusing myself and thanking God that I was going to have this beautiful baby and everything was going to be okay.

Finally, my water broke on my first push. After just two more pushes, my baby was out! I needed no stitches and my little Donovan was in perfect health. He was actually my first baby who didn't have any jaundice, either.

The doctors and nurses performed all sorts of tests and checked him a little bit more carefully because of me being positive for Strep B, but Donovan was absolutely one hundred percent perfect.

Since my husband had been with me throughout the delivery, he went home to take care of our other children. My mother was able to spend the next night with me and baby in the hospital. It was really a special time.

I was sent home the next day and spent New Year's Eve with our new little addition to the family. God is so good!

chapter nine
Full House

Our home was very full now and we decided not to have any more children. Four was definitely more than what we had initially imagined. Along with our ministries, we could see how God was transitioning us. Our family was now complete.

I can't tell you why some of my babies are in heaven, but I can tell you that everything changed when I believed God for more than what the doctors told me and I began to walk in faith and expect my prayers to be answered.

Faith is simple. God doesn't make us do all these things religion has told us we need to do to get God's attention. He simply tells us to trust Him. His Word is truth and it is His will. So if you can get the Word in you and believe what it says, you can walk and live by faith.

> *And without faith it is impossible to please God, because anyone who comes to him must believe that he exists and that he rewards those who earnestly seek him.*
>
> —Hebrews 11:6

The Promised Child

For in the gospel the righteousness of God is revealed—a righteousness that is by faith from first to last, just as it is written: "The righteous will live by faith."

—Romans 1:17

Now faith is confidence in what we hope for and assurance about what we do not see.

—Hebrews 11:1

When I really wanted answers from God, I started to spend more time with Him. Our relationship became important to me. I wanted to know Him and hear Him. I wanted Him to reveal His truth to me.

My husband and I dove into the Word and listened to the teachings that changed our lives. But we didn't just do it once—we still do it every day.

When God answered our prayers with these pregnancies and our beautiful babies, we began to trust and believe Him in every area of our lives. We filled ourselves with healing scriptures the same way we filled ourselves with financial scriptures, overcoming fear scriptures, peace and joy scriptures, love scriptures, marriage, family, etc. God's Word has it all.

We were set free from stress and anxiety. We weren't worried anymore about our health, finances, or daily struggles. God showed us that the dreams in our hearts, and the great destiny we have, are all attainable! He shows us how to dream the impossible and live successfully in every area. If you can make your dreams happen, they aren't big enough. Dreams require God.

Some people have asked me how I'm able to stay at home and raise our children on one income. They see us owning our home and living with all the things we need. But that is God! I wanted to stay at home; we have faith for me to stay at home. When you can pay off your debts and learn to listen to God, He will bring you everything you need and want. He loves us more than we can even imagine and He wants to show the world that we are His beloved children.

I want to share with you some of the life-changing scriptures I began to repeat to myself and get into my heart.

For the mouth speaks what the heart is full of.
—Matthew 12:34

The tongue has the power of life and death, and those who love it will eat its fruit.
—Proverbs 18:21

You must be fully convinced that God's Word is final. *You* have power and authority over your situations. God gave you all authority through Jesus.

And if the Spirit of him who raised Jesus from the dead is living in you, he who raised Christ from the dead will also give life to your mortal bodies because of his Spirit who lives in you.
—Romans 8:11

And as Pastor Gary Keesee has been known to say, "That is the agreement between heaven and earth—that is faith."

The Promised Child

I would read these scriptures out loud to myself, or with my husband, every day when we were waiting to get pregnant, during pregnancy, and even in delivery. I chose these scriptures because they spoke about my situation and gave me hope and confidence as I read them. I found myself filled with joy and greater expectations of what God could do. Then the results followed.

The fruit of your womb will be blessed...
—Deuteronomy 28:4

Children are a heritage from the Lord, offspring a reward from him.
—Psalm 127:3

The Lord will grant you abundant prosperity—in the fruit of your womb...
—Deuteronomy 28:11

...he blesses your children within you.
—Psalm 147:13, ESV

All your children will be taught by the Lord, and great will be their peace.
—Isaiah 54:13

But women will be saved through childbearing—if they continue in faith, love and holiness with propriety.
—I Timothy 2:15

Surprise

None shall lose her young by miscarriage or be barren in your land; I will fulfill the number of your days.
—Exodus 23:26, AMPC

He will love you, bless you, and multiply you. He will also bless the fruit of your womb...
—Deuteronomy 7:13, ESV

Didn't the Lord make you one with your wife? In body and spirit you are his. And what does he want? Godly children from your union.
—Malachi 2:15, NLT

By faith Sarah herself received power to conceive, even when she was past the age, since she considered him faithful who had promised.
—Hebrews 11:11, ESV

He shall... gently lead those who are with young.
—Isaiah 40:11, KJV

Be strong and courageous. Do not be afraid or terrified because of them, for the Lord your God goes with you; he will never leave you nor forsake you.
—Deuteronomy 31:6

For he will command his angels concerning you to guard you in all your ways
—Psalm 91:11

The Promised Child

...fully convinced that God was able to do what he had promised.
—Romans 4:21, ESV

This is the confidence we have in approaching God: that if we ask anything according to his will, he hears us. And if we know that he hears us—whatever we ask—we know that we have what we asked of him.
—1 John 5:14–15

This day I call the heavens and the earth as witnesses against you that I have set before you life and death, blessings and curses. Now choose life, so that you and your children may live...

—Deuteronomy 30:19

Truly I tell you, if anyone says to this mountain, 'Go, throw yourself into the sea,' and does not doubt in their heart but believes that what they say will happen, it will be done for them. Therefore I tell you, whatever you ask for in prayer, believe that you have received it, and it will be yours.

—Mark 11:23–24

These are just a few of God's great promises for us. His Word has the power to convince your heart and grow your faith—and it is power, so speak it out loud! God created the world by speaking it into existence.

Last but not least, I encourage you to worship. Sometimes when you don't understand your situations or cannot see the next step, just begin to praise and worship God.

Surprise

...for the joy of the Lord is your strength.

—Nehemiah 8:10

You can have peace and strength in trying situations. You set the ambiance in a room and in your heart when you bring God's praise into it.

God gave me a vision one day during a worship service. It was a vision of Jesus standing in a circle with some children holding their hands and dancing. My heart immediately told me that those were my kids in heaven.

Through Christ we already have the victory to overcome (1 Corinthians 15:57). That means that if we trust in Jesus, whatever may come our way, we don't have to be afraid, for He has equipped us with all that we need to fulfill His Word. I have learned that everyone isn't going to agree with the way you talk or conduct yourself, but your testimony speaks louder than any good sermon. Our lives reflect the Good News of Jesus Christ.

I can do all this through him who gives me strength.

—Philippians 4:13

I would rather be someone who encourages others and speaks life into every situation than someone who just brings people down with negativity and complaining. There's too much of that in this world.

I have hope, and I will stand on it and share it!

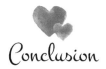

Conclusion

I can say today that I'm thankful to be able to speak to so many women about my testimony and encourage everyone in their faith. I have seen many answered prayers and miraculous births because of it!

For all my family and friends who have witnessed these events firsthand, God has touched you as well. We can't deny the miracle-working power of God.

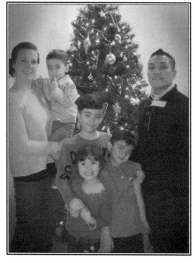

Friends, it is so important for you to have healing, restoration, and hope. I pray that this book has encouraged and inspired you, and I pray that faith is growing in your heart.

If you haven't invited Christ into your heart yet, there's nothing holding you back. God has every answer and can fill every need you have. He is always there for you and has great plans for you. Please make Him number one in your life.

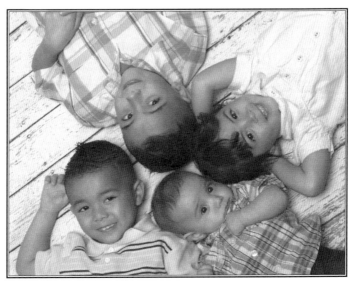

I encourage you to connect with me. If you need someone who will understand what you may be going through, or have gone through, or if you need someone to stand in faith with you today, please reach out to me by email: c.amoyo@gmail.com

Blessings to you all.

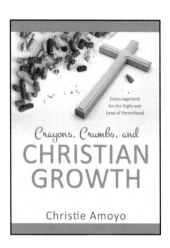

Crayons, Crumbs, and Christian Growth
ISBN: 978-1-4866-1714-2

Parenting children is a wonderful blessing that comes with great challenges. As you navigate the waters of parenthood, it can be easy to feel disconnected from life and your faith. You may think you are alone on this journey, and you may be frustrated trying to meet the demands all around you.

But these years can be the greatest of your life—years in which God shows you how real He is, how faith actually works, and how you can enjoy the blessings He's given you. In *Crayons, Crumbs, and Christian Growth*, Christie shares about how the trials and treasures of parenting her own children has taught her so much about who God is.